Your Tube: A Guide to Nutrition Through a Feeding Tube

Your Tube

A guide to nutrition
through a feeding tube

LINA BREIK

Advanced Accredited Practising Dietitian

Typesetting by BookPOD
Cover artwork by Kathryn Lean

ISBN: 978-0-6459873-0-0 (pbk)
ISBN: 978-0-6459873-1-7 (e-book)

NATIONAL
LIBRARY
OF AUSTRALIA

A catalogue record for this
book is available from the
National Library of Australia

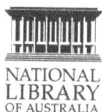

"Nutrition goes beyond medication; it stands as a human right, a manifestation of love, a reflection of cultural identity and an important aspect of our social connections. This essence remains unchanged even when delivered through a feeding tube."

– Lina Breik

Contents

Foreword

OUR WORLD IS NOT BEAUTIFUL because we're all the same. Our world is beautiful because we're all different. In 2023, it's estimated that we are 8 billion different lives roaming this planet. As humanity, diversity is who we are.

When we empower each other to be different, we are all richer for it. At the heart of healthcare, this is a large part of what the work is all about – empowering each other to live our best lives while celebrating our own unique selves.

And an important part of a best life is good nutrition. It is the fuel, the foundation, that allows us to be who we are. With the right nutrition, everything has the potential to fall into place. But we are not all the same in the way we access nutrition. For some, it's with a knife and fork. For some, it's with chopsticks. For some, it's with hands. For some, it's soft foods. For some, it's with a tube.

This is not new. Feeding tubes are said to date back around 3500 years to the times of ancient Egyptians. They've been around for a long time. Over those 3500 years, many human beings have and continue to use feeding tubes. Although it's a relatively simple piece of ingenuity, a feeding tube is not without its little intricacies. That's where a guide comes in handy.

It's not just about the technical know-how though. It was once said that the biggest mistake is to separate our physical self from our spirit when it comes to good health and wellness. So, it's important to talk about matters of the spirit when we dig into thriving with a feeding tube.

That's what Lina's passion has brought to life in *Your Tube*. It's a book aimed at celebrating you and empowering you to live your best life, while acknowledging your value in the rich tapestry of our society.

Dr Dinesh Palipana OAM
Leading disability advocate, lawyer and emergency doctor

"The one thing that all people with disabilities have in common when it comes to nutrition is the right for their individual nutrition needs to be upheld."

– Dr Dinesh Palipana OAM

Introduction

Empowering yourself

IN A WORLD WHERE OUR bodies constantly undergo internal and external changes, it's crucial to foster a sense of control and understanding. There is a wealth of options when it comes to nurturing wellbeing, and it's within your power to navigate this path with knowledge and intention.

Welcome to *Your Tube: A guide to nutrition through a feeding tube*. This book aims to empower individuals who are reliant on feeding tubes to confidently navigate the intricate world of nutrition. By understanding the fundamentals of a feeding tube and recognising that nutrition through a tube can still be delivered with love and flexibility – as it is for those without feeding tubes – a tube-fed person can overcome their fears and jump into the driver's seat to advocate for themselves and ensure their optimal wellbeing.

This book is designed for the adult tube-fed person who is living at home and is medically stable. *It should not be taken as a substitute for professional medical or dietetic advice as every individual's medical condition and nutritional requirements are unique*, but rather as a means to empower tube-fed adults with knowledge they may not have had the capacity to absorb before leaving hospital. A recent scientific publication defined individualised nutrition care for tube-fed people in the community as inclusive of "discussions of the type of tube, method of administration (pump, bolus, intermittent), feeding regimen and the types of feed". The authors also emphasised that counselling on options available "can empower them to make choices and enable them to alert healthcare professionals when issues arise that could be managed by altering aspects of feed choice" (Holdoway et al. 2022:4). And that is exactly what this book has been designed to do: empower you with the knowledge of options.

Medical jargon like 'anthropometry' has been purposely used so that you can understand the things your dietitian or other health care providers say. Whether you are about to have a feeding tube inserted, care for someone who has an existing feeding tube or are seeking to enhance your existing knowledge, these pages hold the key to unlocking your full potential.

Now, let's take a brief journey through each chapter.

Chapter 1, 'Exploring the abundance of options', delves into the myriad choices you may encounter as you strive for optimal health. From different formulas to feeding regimen options, this chapter equips you with the knowledge to make informed decisions, enabling you to customise your journey according to your unique needs. By understanding the options available to you, you can embark on a transformative journey towards a healthier and more fulfilling life.

In Chapter 2, 'Understanding anthropometry', we delve into the significance of body measurements and how they reflect your overall health. By comprehending the subtle shifts in your physicality, you can track progress and make necessary adjustments to your feeding tube nutrition, developing an appreciation for the remarkable nature of your body.

Chapter 3, 'Nurturing clinical wellbeing', explores the importance of monitoring potential red flags and recognising their significance in maintaining overall health. By arming yourself with this knowledge, you become a proactive participant in your wellbeing.

Chapter 4, 'Nourishing your body', takes you on a voyage through the realm of nutrition requirements. With a focus on fluid, protein, calories and micronutrients, we uncover the foundational elements of nutrition, ensuring that you nourish yourself in the most effective and sustainable way possible.

Chapter 5, 'Rising above challenges', has helpful tips for dealing with common feeding tube issues, including things like preventing blockages by staying on top of regular maintenance and taking quick action if your tube ever gets dislodged. The key here is being proactive and staying ahead of the game.

Chapter 6, 'Supporting the spirit', acknowledges the emotional dimensions of your wellbeing, particularly within the context of the feeding tube experience. This chapter discusses the complexities of the emotional journey, offering guidance and support to those navigating this unique path.

Throughout this book, you will find valuable insights, practical tips and guidance to empower you on your journey towards wellbeing. Embrace this opportunity to take control, explore your options, write specific questions you have for your dietitian or other healthcare providers, and nurture your body, mind and spirit. Commit yourself to embarking on a transformative path towards a healthier and more vibrant life with you in the driver's seat.

Chapter 1

Exploring the abundance of options

HAVING A FEEDING TUBE CAN indeed be a life-altering experience, but it's important to recognise that it can often bring about several positive changes that offer individuals a second chance at life. A tube-fed adult I worked with recently said, "It's given me a second chance at being an energetic mother to my five children plus being able to complete my doctoral studies."

As the person with the feeding tube, you are at the centre of your care team. You play the most crucial role as the driver of your own care. It is your body, your health and your decisions that matter. You have the power to take control of your feeding tube journey, making choices that align with your unique needs and preferences. You might wonder, "What options do I have?" Rest assured, there are a multitude of options available to you. Let's explore some of these options and embrace the freedom they provide.

FORMULA

There are two overarching options for the formula you can be on:

1. Commercial formulas.

2. Homemade blended formulas.

Commercial formulas

There are a wide range of formula choices available to you. In Australia, the main formula companies are Abbott, Nutricia, Fresenius Kabi and Nestle. Jump on their websites, research their products and consult your dietitian about any potential switches you are considering and the reasons behind them. The ultimate decision rests with you and your dietitian to determine what works best for your body and preferences.

Commercial formulas differ in several ways. If you believe that your bowel habits, weight, nutrition goals, activity levels, energy levels, quality of life and social activity participation have not reached their maximum potential, it might be time to contemplate switching formulas. Consider these questions:

Do you have a big day of activities and need extra calories? Do your bowel habits keep you going often to the toilet?

Here are some formula characteristics to consider with your dietitian:

1. **Calorie concentration**
   1.0kcal/ml is the lowest calorie content formula. 2.0kcal/ml formulas have double the calorie content in the same amount of fluid. For example, for those on fluid restrictions or those who prefer less volume delivery throughout the day, the 2.0kcal/ml formulas are a great option for providing enough nutrition with not much volume.

2. **Fibre content**
   Fibre is necessary for bowel health. If you aren't on a fibre-containing formula, consult your dietitian. Unless you have a gastrointestinal condition that contradicts fibre in your diet, switching to a fibre-containing formula for bowel health is undisputed in the scientific literature (Elia et al. 2008).

3. **Electrolyte content**
   For those with kidney disease or who need a low sodium / low potassium formula for any other reason, these are a great option.

4. **Pre-digested vs whole proteins**
   The majority of formulas consist of whole proteins but if you need a pre-digested formula, for example, due

to pancreas issues, pre-digested protein-containing formulas may be a better option for you.

5. **Disease-specific formulas**

   Specialised enteral formulas are created for specific medical conditions like diabetes, wound healing, kidney disease and liver failure. These formulas have unique nutrient compositions targeted for each condition (e.g. high protein for wound healing). However, a standard whole protein formula can often meet the nutritional needs of people with these conditions.

6. **Plant-based formulas**

   These are formulas derived from plant-based ingredients such as soy, rice and peas and are free of animal products and common allergens. These are suitable for vegans or those who wish to opt for a more environmentally friendly option (Griffen et al. 2023).

7. **125–200ml packaged formulas vs 500–1000ml**

   If the current 1L bottle you are using is too heavy to carry during social outings, you may want to investigate formulas packaged in a more travel-friendly manner (i.e. 200ml or 125ml bottles or cans).

8. **Bottle capped vs spike capped**

   If you have arthritis, opting for a formula with a screwable bottle cap rather than a spike cap can make a significant difference in terms of ease and comfort for you to deliver your own feeds.

9. **Commercially made 'whole food' or 'real food' formulas**

   These formulas typically aim to include minimally processed ingredients and maintain the nutritional integrity of the whole foods they are made from. But keep in mind that the quality and nutritional profile of these products can vary widely.

Formula adjustments can greatly improve your experience with a feeding tube. The empowering aspect is that, together with your dietitian, you have the ability to select a formula that perfectly aligns with your requirements and also with the way you want to live your life.

Homemade blended formulas

It's important to note that homemade blended tube feeding (BTF) formulas are a viable option as well. In fact, more and more tube-fed adults are opting for BTF whether for cost, social, personal or formula intolerance reasons. A recent survey conducted in Australia and New Zealand found that 40% of home tube feeding hospital services report their patients using BTF for a portion or all of their nutrition needs (Flood et al. 2021). So, it's happening!

If fresh whole foods are used – blended to the right consistency and with vigilant food hygiene practices – it can be a nourishing path to go down. For some people, homemade BTF provides social inclusivity at the dinner table, as they are often able to have what everyone else is eating. Others find it more cost-effective or prefer it as it's a more natural option (Hurt et al. 2015; Walia et al. 2017). Even though it is debatable whether commercial formula or BTF is superior, you have the right and autonomy to choose BTF if that is what you want.

Seek the assistance of a dietitian experienced in feeding tubes and BTF to develop nourishing recipes and ensure proper blending. Refer to Appendix 1 for a brief overview of homemade BTF and what it entails.

Remember to consult with your dietitian before making any changes. Determining the best formula for your specific needs and circumstances involves a myriad of aspects such as your medical goals, nutrition goals, gastrointestinal anatomy and more. This shouldn't be a one-size-fits-all or a set-and-forget approach. Your nutrition should grow and change with you.

REGIMEN

In addition to the formula, you have the power to determine your feeding regimen mode, method and schedule. This decision depends on your medical condition, surgical history, if you are on any time-specific medications like insulin and your capacity to manage larger volumes of formula. Let's explore your regimen options in more detail with examples.

Mode

There are three modes to consider:

1. Continuous.
2. Bolus.
3. Combination.

Continuous feeding involves the gradual and consistent infusion of nutrition, either spanning 24 hours or for a specific period during the day or night such as 10- or 12-hour feeding intervals. The latter can sometimes be termed 'intermittent feeding mode'. The rate of formula administration is typically around 100ml/hr or more, tailored to your digestive system's capacity.

On the other hand, bolus feeding follows a pattern of 15–20-minute feed times occurring two to six times a day, with each session comprising approximately 250ml (a cup) or more of formula. The volume per bolus is highly individualised, depending on your digestive system's tolerance. This feeding method closely emulates a mealtime eating pattern.

A combination of these methods is also possible. Your feeding regimen should adapt to fit your life, not the other way around. So, if you enjoy hiking, you can adjust your feeding regimen to accommodate your active days by having a 15-minute bolus through a syringe at midday for some energy for the hike, and then infusing the rest of your required formula amount via pump continuously once you get home for a 10-hour period. Likewise, on lazy Sundays, you might opt for a pump and continuous feeding in front of the TV. Flexibility is key, and you have the ability to customise your regimen to your unique circumstances.

Method

When it comes to the method of delivering the chosen mode, you have a few different options to choose from:

1. Feeding pump method.
2. Drip method (sometimes referred to as gravity drip).
3. Syringe method.

Pumps offer convenience and automated delivery, allowing precise control over the rate and duration of feedings. They are more appropriate for those who have had surgery on their stomach or other organs of the digestive system as they allow a slower infusion of nutrition over a set period of time. For example, if someone needs 1200ml of formula per day through a pump, that can be a continuous 120ml/hr over a ten-hour period during the day or overnight, or bolus as 100ml/hr for four hours three times a day via pump (0700–1100, 1300–1700, 1900–2300).

The drip method or gravity drip is where gravity controls the speed of formula dropping into your feeding tube and is often at a gentler pace than pump. This would involve a giving set (the line that connects from the formula bottle to your feeding tube) and just allowing gravity to drip the formula down. The rate can be controlled to some extent as the giving set required for this method has a roller clamp to adjust the rate.

On the other hand, some individuals prefer the simplicity, speed and portability of using syringes (often 60ml in size) and allowing the feed to go down with gravity. This would take 15–20 minutes per bolus mimicking mealtimes and can look like this: 250ml of formula at 0800, 1200, 1400, 1700, 2000 (totalling 1250ml of formula in 24 hours).

To summarise which method can be used for what mode, check out this table:

	CONTINUOUS	BOLUS	COMBINATION
PUMP	X	X	X
DRIP	X	X	X
SYRINGE		X	X

Discuss all options with your dietitian and determine which one aligns best with your preferences and lifestyle.

Schedule

Flexibility also extends to your feeding schedule. You have the autonomy to decide when to have your meals, and it doesn't have to be at the same time every day.

Unless you have specific medical requirements, such as being dependent on insulin for blood glucose control, you can adjust your feeding time to fit your daily routine and activities. Embrace the freedom to make each day different and adapt your feeding schedule accordingly. Those without a feeding tube definitely don't eat at the exact same time each day!

Some tube-fed adults appreciate the volume-based approach, where they consider the total amount of formula needed for the day and then find ways to incorporate it into their daily routine. For instance, if you require 1200ml of formula daily and have social outings planned, you can opt to bolus feed 300ml through a syringe four times during the day. Alternatively, if you are busy away from home, you can temporarily set the feeding aside and resume it by pumping the remaining amount when you return home in the evening. This flexible approach allows for seamless integration of feeding into various activities throughout the day.

The goal is a feeding regimen that changes based on your needs, such as weekdays when you're mainly at home, work or school compared to weekends when you want to be more active and social. It's possible to create a regimen that caters to both scenarios, is supported by your dietitian and is led by you.

Now, what about overnight feeding? This is a common question. Overnight feeding disrupts the natural circadian rhythm (or 'body clock'), which is designed for wakefulness and nutrition during the day and sleep at night. Scientific research shows that overnight nutrition, demonstrated in the shift worker population, can have negative impacts on blood glucose control, weight and heart health (Torquati et al. 2017). While some cases necessitate overnight feeding, such as hospital patients or those on certain medications, shifting to daytime feeding is advisable for overall long-term health.

On the following pages are three examples illustrating real-life feeding regimens that are very different and have each been crafted carefully by a tube-fed adult and their dietitian. Remember to consult your dietitian first before making any changes to your regimen.

Example 1: Bolus pump feeding during the day

MEAL	TIME	TUBE FEED	WATER AMOUNT
Breakfast (400ml formula)	0600–until complete	130ml/hr	Medications with 60ml water before and after. 100ml after feed stops.
Break			
Lunch (400ml formula)	1200–until complete	130ml/hr	Medications with 60ml water before and after. 100ml after feed stops.
Break			
Dinner (400ml formula)	1800–until complete	130ml/hr	Medications with 60ml water before and after. 100ml after feed stops.

Your Tube

Example 2: Bolus syringe feeding four times a day

TIME	TUBE FEED	MEAL THROUGH THE MOUTH	WATER AMOUNT
0730	188ml	—	50ml before 50ml after
Morning tea	—	As desired + 250ml tea/ coffee	
1100	188ml	—	50ml before 50ml after
1500	188ml	—	50ml before 50ml after
Afternoon tea	—	As desired + 250ml tea/ coffee	
1800	188ml	—	50ml before 50ml after
2000	—	—	200ml

Example 3: Continuous pump feeding in the evening

TIME	TUBE FEED	MEDICATION	WATER AMOUNT
1500	—	Parkinson's disease medication*	50ml before 125ml after
1700	200ml/hr	—	100ml before
2200	200ml/hr	—	100ml after
2300	—	Parkinson's disease medication*	50ml before 125ml after

*For this client, their Parkinson's disease medication needs to be taken on an empty stomach. This applies to tube feeding too! Make sure you chat with your doctor and dietitian about potential medication-nutrient interactions.

Transitioning

Transitioning from pump feeding to bolus syringe feeding (and vice versa) can happen progressively over a week or so, or cold turkey the next day. The best approach for you is that determined by you and your dietitian. Factors such as your gastrointestinal anatomy, your tolerance to larger volumes of formula and what equipment you have available at home play a role in how quickly you transition from one schedule or mode or formula to another.

Intolerance to a feeding mode, method, schedule or formula can present as (not exclusive) bloating, nausea, vomiting and/or a drastic change in bowel habits. More on this in Chapter 5 but remember that tube feeding shouldn't be a set-and-forget situation. It can and should flex with your life.

TUBE

During the initial insertion of your feeding tube, you might not have been able to participate in decisions around what type of tube went in due to your hospitalisation and health condition. However, now that you are well and back home (or about to be discharged from hospital), you have the opportunity to have a say in selecting certain characteristics for your next tube change. Familiarising yourself with these tube characteristics will empower you to make an informed decision. The more you understand about your feeding tube, the more in control you can be. Let's delve into tube characteristics and explore your options.

Where it starts

Short-term feeding tubes are the ones that usually start at the nose (i.e. nasogastric and nasojejunal). These tubes are often inserted for four- to six-week periods and then need to be either removed or replaced with a new one. Long-term tubes last for a year or more if well cared for and they start at the abdomen (i.e. gastrostomy or jejunostomy).

Where it ends

The placement of the feeding tube, whether in the stomach or small intestine, depends on factors such as your underlying condition that necessitated the tube and your gastrointestinal anatomy. Generally, this decision is made by your care team during your hospital stay. However, don't forget to ask about where your tube ends before you leave the hospital. Tubes that end in the stomach (i.e. tubes that have the word 'gastric' or 'gastrostomy' in them) can generally deliver larger volumes than those that end in the small intestine (i.e. tubes that have the word 'jejunal' or 'duodenal' or 'jejunostomy' in them) (Kong and Singh 2008). However, this doesn't mean if you have a jejunal ending tube that you are fully restricted to being attached to a continuous pump feed with a tiny amount of 50ml/hr! Some people's small intestines can manage large volumes of formula similar to a stomach, and there is scientific research to support that it is safe (Parrish and Bridges 2019). It's just about trial and error, working with your digestive system and with your dietitian.

How was it inserted?

The method of tube insertion is also determined by your care team. It can be done at the bedside, such as with short-term tubes inserted through the nose, or through endoscopy, radiology or surgery for longer-term tubes. A percutaneous **endoscopic** gastrostomy (PEG) tube and a **radiologically** inserted gastrostomy (RIG) tube both have their insertion method in their name (notice the words in bold). Jejunostomies (JEJ) are surgically inserted and sewn in place, and they end in the second part of the small intestine (i.e. the jejunum). If you don't have a tube as yet but will be getting one soon, know that each method has different requirements for anaesthesia and length of stay in hospital. PEGs can be done as a day procedure, for example. Discuss what would be best for your specific condition with your doctor early.

Button or dangler?

In the case of long-term feeding tubes that protrude from the abdomen, you can choose between a button tube or a dangler tube. Button tubes do not hang freely; they stop at the level of your abdomen, allowing them to be hidden under clothing. Button tubes need to be connected to an extension set and then to the feeding syringe or pump. Dangler tubes, on the other hand, hang outside the abdomen and require less equipment to operate (no need for an extension set), but they can be accidentally tugged on and dislodged. It's important to weigh the pros and cons of both options and discuss them with your care team to make the appropriate decision for you.

Diameter of the tube

Feeding tubes also come in different diameter sizes, referred to as 'French size'. This indicates the outer diameter of the tube. The size can be found on the tubing itself and is abbreviated as 'Fr'. Tubes with a larger diameter (typically above 14 Fr) are more beneficial for homemade blends to accommodate for the potential variability in thickness of the blends.

Additionally, you'll also find the brand of a tube written on its tubing which is useful to note for two reasons:

1. Most manufacturers have a customer care line to provide support for troubleshooting equipment or tube-related issues.
2. You know the brand to purchase a spare tube or two to keep at home in case of an emergency where you can take your spare tube to the closest emergency department for replacement or insertion.

Anchoring device

Anchoring devices are those that hold a feeding tube in its place. Here are various ways in which feeding tubes can be anchored in place:

-   Short-term tubes (i.e. nasogastric and nasojejunal):
    -   Adhesive tape on the cheek.
    -   A bridle retention device. Bridles consist of a soft, flexible loop made of medical-grade material that is inserted through one nostril and exits through the other (Lynch et al. 2018). This can be very helpful as it

reduces the risk of the tube being pulled out accidentally during a shower or sleep. It's not for everybody though and does come with risks.

Remember to check the centimetre marking of the tube at the tip of your nose daily and ask your doctor or dietitian "What's holding my tube in its place?" and "What should the centimetre marking at my nose tip be?"

- Longer-term tubes (i.e. PEG, RIG, JEJ):
  - A balloon.
  - A collapsible flange.
  - A rigid flange.
  - Surgical sutures.

The specific anchoring device for long-term tubes depends on factors such as the insertion technique, whether it's an initial tube or a replacement, and your doctor's preference. Among these options, balloon anchored tubes are the most convenient since they can be replaced without requiring a hospital visit. You would need to regularly check the balloon volume of water (usually around 3–10ml), typically on a weekly basis or as determined by your specific needs. Tubes with a collapsible flange can be removed by pulling, while rigid flanged tubes should only be removed at endoscopy.

The knowledge is yours now. Keep it in mind for when it's time for a tube replacement. Discuss each feature with your doctor and decide what works best for you.

In terms of when you should get a tube replaced, generally speaking, any kinks, cracks, discolouration, sedimentation and/or leakage should warrant a change.

Feeding tube ports

Feeding tube ports are pretty much the doorway that connects feeding tubes from the outside to the inside of your digestive system. A tube might come with just one port that handles everything – formula, medication and water flushes. Others may have multiple feeding ports – one for formula, one for medications, one for access to the small intestine, one for access to the balloon anchoring device, etc. Take note of how many ports your tube has and ask your dietitian what each one is for.

The other key thing about ports is whether they are ENFit ended. ENFit is an international standard for ports in feeding tubes, separate from those used for intravenous tubes. This standard ensures proper and secure fitting of feeding tube equipment to the feeding tube. While not all tubes have ENFit ended ports, all feeding equipment is ENFit ended. So, in this instance, using an adaptor is necessary to allow ENFit equipment to be used. If your tube lacks an ENFit ended port, requesting one during the next tube change can greatly improve equipment fit, minimising leaks and enhancing security.

EQUIPMENT

What type of equipment do I need is a question that pops up a lot. The answer really depends on two main things:

1. What kind of regimen you are on.
2. What kind of tube you have.

Instead of getting into the nitty-gritty details of every single piece of equipment (as it can differ from one company to another), let's keep it simple with a table that highlights the main equipment used and when they might come in handy. Please note the terms in the table might not match what's used everywhere. And don't forget, it's always a good idea to chat with your dietitian before you go out and buy any extra gear for your feeding tube setup.

EQUIPMENT	WHAT IS IT?	WHEN IS IT NEEDED?
Giving set	Connection from the formula to your feeding tube. They have various features such as a medication y-port, a gravity drip chamber, a roller clamp or a bottle/spike top.	The exact features you need in your giving sets depends on your formula and feeding method.
Extension set	Connection from your feeding tube to the giving set for pump feeding or to the syringe for bolus feeding. They come as 'right angled' or 'straight' connectors and also come in different centimetre sizes.	For those who have button tubes.
ENFit transition adaptor	Use to connect a non-ENFit feeding tube to ENFit ended equipment.	For those who have a non-ENFit ended feeding tube.

EQUIPMENT	WHAT IS IT?	WHEN IS IT NEEDED?
Syringe	Come in various sizes such as 10ml, 20ml, 60ml, etc.	Can be used for water flushes, medication administration and formula delivery.
pH strips	Strips used to test the pH of the fluid drawn out of your body from the feeding tube.	Used for gastrostomy tubes to check that the tube is actually in the stomach.
Enteral backpack	A backpack with specific compartments designed for enteral feeding equipment.	Used for pump feeding on the go or can be used for syringe bolus feeding to keep everything organised in a dedicated backpack.
Pump	An electronic pump specifically designed for tube feeding.	Pump feeding.
Pump stand or pole	A stand or pole to rest your pump on.	Pump feeding.

EQUIPMENT	WHAT IS IT?	WHEN IS IT NEEDED?
Bolus holder	A clamp that holds a syringe upright, freeing your arms during bolus feeding.	Syringe bolus feeding.
Empty containers	Can come in various sizes and usually sterile packaged.	For decanting formula into a smaller or larger container. For storing powder formula or homemade blends.
Adhesive skin tape	Skin-friendly tape.	To tape nasal feeding tubes to your cheek so they stay out of the way when not in use.
Gastrostomy belt	A specifically designed belt used to tuck in your dangler feeding tube.	For dangler feeding tubes so they stay out of the way when not in use.

Additionally, there are several innovative feeding tube accessories created by individuals who either use feeding tubes themselves or care for someone who relies on them. These accessories can make life with a feeding tube more enjoyable and easier.

Explore the following as a start:

- FreeArm – www.freearmcare.com
- A Simple Patch – www.asimplepatch.com
- Tubie Fun – www.tubiefun.com.au
- Tubie Love – www.tubielove.com

CARE TEAM

As the one in control, you have the authority to assemble your care team: a group of individuals who will offer the support, guidance and expertise necessary for your feeding tube journey. When selecting care team members, consider involving professionals such as doctors, dietitians, nurses and even speech pathologists and physiotherapists, depending on your specific needs.

Trust and compatibility are crucial factors when choosing individuals who will be involved in your home tube feeding journey. If you feel the need to hide information from your care team, such as putting your grandmother's blended pumpkin soup through the tube, it may be time to consider finding different clinicians who can better support you. Seek clinicians who value independence, autonomy, outside-the-box thinking and flexibility. It's also important to ensure that the care team you choose are experienced and well-versed in feeding tube management in the community.

Ideally, your care team should include a nurse with feeding tube experience who you can reach out to for troubleshooting tube issues and a dietitian specialised in feeding tube nutrition who you can consult regarding bowel, weight or other nutritional concerns. Do not hesitate to ask your existing clinician if they are experienced in guiding people with feeding tubes and then act accordingly. It is your right to ask, and having an experienced team by your side will make your life much easier. Your care team should be a source of support and understanding, ensuring that your unique needs are met.

YOUR CIRCLE OF INFLUENCE

Your circle of influence extends to the aspects within your control, such as the composition of your care team, your chosen formula and feeding regimen, and whether you use a pump or syringe and a button or dangler. These elements directly impact your experience with the feeding tube.

However, it's important to recognise that there are factors beyond your control, including the underlying circumstances that necessitate the need for a feeding tube, the location where the tube ends, the insertion method and the physical positioning of the tube.

By focusing on what you can control, you can enhance your feeding tube journey. While you are at home and medically stable, take the opportunity to explore different formulas and find the one that best suits your nutritional requirements. Fine-tune your feeding regimen to align with your daily schedule and activities. Remember, you are the one in control so feel empowered to make decisions that prioritise your overall wellbeing.

Consider these self-reflection questions to assess if changes are needed:

- Does my current formula provide me with sufficient energy to go about my day the way I want to?
- How does my feeding routine affect my day-to-day activities?
- Does my feeding regimen restrict my ability to participate in social activities?
- How can I plan my tube feeding to ensure I can attend as many social outings as I would like to in a week?
- Does my care team support and respect the choices I suggest regarding my feeding tube nutrition or do I find myself hiding information from them?

In the upcoming chapter, we will delve into anthropometric indicators that you should be vigilant about and highlight when it is necessary to bring them to the attention of your dietitian.

Remember that you have the ability to chart your own path, and the choices you make along the way are significant.

Chapter 2

Understanding anthropometry

WHEN IT COMES TO YOUR feeding tube journey, understanding anthropometry, the measurement of your body and its changes, is crucial. By closely monitoring your body's response to tube-fed nutrition, you can identify any significant weight loss or gain, assess muscle and fat stores, and even consider the impact of water weight. Let's explore these aspects in more detail.

UNINTENTIONAL WEIGHT LOSS

Unintentional weight loss is a matter of concern for individuals, whether they have feeding tubes or not, as it may indicate inadequate nutrition or other underlying problems. However, it's essential to understand that not all weight loss is necessarily problematic. The key is in the word unintentional. 'Clinically significant' unintentional weight loss is defined as a loss of 5% or more within a month (Stajkovic et al. 2011). Your dietitian can assist you in determining whether the unintentional weight loss you're experiencing falls within that definition, considering your specific circumstances. At times, the amount of weight loss may not meet that specific criteria but can still be relevant and worrisome to you. Consider factors like your initial weight, height and nutritional goals to establish a meaningful threshold for weight loss that requires action. By establishing this baseline, you can identify when weight loss exceeds the expected range and take appropriate measures.

UNINTENTIONAL WEIGHT GAIN

On the other hand, it's important to also note that unintentional weight gain can occur throughout your feeding tube journey. Unlike individuals who consume food orally, those relying on tubes do not have the ability to regulate their intake or control the number of calories consumed in a day based on appetite, hunger, feelings of nausea, etc. Consequently, progressive weight gain resulting from a consistent and constant calorie intake can become a significant issue.

Unintentional weight gain can have implications for your skin integrity and overall health, and mobility becomes more challenging, limiting your activity (Zheng et al. 2017).

Your dietitian can assist you in identifying a healthy weight range and help you understand when weight gain becomes a concern. Nonetheless, it's important to remember that you know your body best.

Communicate your ideal weight to your dietitian and work together towards that goal. Strategies your dietitian may suggest to stop unnecessary progressive weight gain include reducing the volume of formula you receive while simultaneously adding a multivitamin tablet and protein powder scoops. This way, you can lower your calorie intake without compromising your intake of essential micronutrients and protein. Micronutrients play a vital role in overall bodily functions and protein is crucial for maintaining muscle mass, so it's important not to compromise on those aspects when reducing overall calorie intake.

Here is an example of a 36-year-old gentleman who had an unfortunate car accident that resulted in a traumatic brain injury. He was in hospital for five months and was 85kg on hospital discharge. Six months later, his weight went up to 105kg. Transferring him from chair to bed became very difficult for his support carers. He developed a pressure injury on his buttocks and was not in good shape.

This gentleman's tube feeding regimen was six boluses of 125ml bottle formula (2.4kcal/ml), providing 7.5MJ, 1800 calories and 71g protein. To achieve weight loss, his calorie intake was reduced by 2.1MJ or 500 calories. His regimen became four bottles of 125ml formula with six scoops of protein powder mixed with water flushes and a multivitamin, providing 5MJ and 84g protein. Six months later, he was down to 78kg, a healthy weight for his height.

Remember, though, not all weight gain is due to calorie intake. Rapid weight gain may be due to medication side effects or water weight changes in the body. Your dietitian and doctor can help you differentiate when the weight gain is water versus fat.

MUSCLE MASS

Assessing muscle mass is another important aspect of anthropometry. Dietitians are trained to utilise validated tools and techniques to evaluate your body composition. There are eight muscle sites that are involved in a physical malnutrition assessment (Detsky et al. 1987). This assessment empowers you and your dietitian to make informed decisions regarding your nutritional requirements, particularly in terms of protein intake to support muscle health and overall wellbeing. Preserving your muscle mass is of utmost importance for maintaining strength and quality of life.

Protein is a key nutrient involved in muscle mass maintenance. If your muscle mass is at risk, your dietitian may use a higher protein formula or recommend protein powder scoops to be mixed with water flushes or added to your homemade blends. Another approach is to switch to a bolus style feeding regimen, as research indicates that our bodies absorb protein more effectively when consumed as 20–30g in a single meal at intervals during the day (Bauer et al. 2013). Additionally, shifting from overnight to daytime feeds can be beneficial for muscle mass, as the body is more metabolically active during the day, facilitating protein utilisation and muscle building.

Your dietitian will be able to provide personalised protein recommendations based on your individual requirements.

WATER WEIGHT

Water weight, also referred to as fluid retention or oedema, is an important consideration in anthropometry. The human body has the ability to retain or release water, resulting in temporary weight fluctuations. Various factors such as hydration levels, hormonal changes, kidney function and underlying medical conditions like heart failure can influence water retention.

In the case of excessive water weight retention, your doctor may recommend a fluid intake restriction. This may require significant adjustments to your feeding regimen, including the amount of formula or water flushes you consume, so let your dietitian know of any fluid intake restrictions.

On the other hand, you may be showing signs of dehydration, in which case, your doctor or dietitian may suggest increasing water intake. You and your dietitian can collaborate to devise an improved regimen, incorporating additional water flushes or opting for a different formula that has a lower concentration, resulting in more fluid intake for the same calorific value. Signs of dehydration to look out for will be discussed in detail in Chapter 4.

Throughout your feeding tube journey, anthropometric measurements serve as valuable indicators of your body's response to the tube feeding process. By closely monitoring weight changes, assessing muscle and fat stores, and considering the impact of water weight, you and your care team can identify any concerning trends and take appropriate action.

In the next chapter, we will explore additional clinical signs and symptoms that warrant attention. By being vigilant and proactive, you can address any potential complications or issues early on, potentially avoiding a hospital admission.

Chapter 3

Nurturing clinical wellbeing

CLINICAL WELLBEING ENCOMPASSES VARIOUS ASPECTS. In this chapter, we will explore the clinical signs and symptoms related to stoma and tube health, digestive health, stool characteristics, medication considerations, as well as skin, hair, nail and eye health. By keeping a close eye on these indicators, you can ensure that your feeding tube journey is optimised for your overall wellbeing.

STOMA HEALTH

For those who have a long-term feeding tube like a PEG, RIG or JEJ, the stoma serves as the entry point for the tube into your body. It is a purposely created hole.

Here are four key things to keep in mind when it comes to stomas:

1. **Daily cleansing**

   Cleanse the stoma daily using warm water, soap and a fresh cloth. Just like brushing your teeth, it should become part of your routine to keep the area clean and dry.

2. **Regular evaluation**

   Regular evaluation of the stoma by a doctor or nurse is essential to ensure proper healing and functionality.

3. **A coin width away!**

   Remember to have a coin width (or 2–5mm) distance between your abdomen and the external skin disc or flange, and always keep that area dry. This can help prevent any pressure sores from forming in that area, as well as prevent any moisture from building and creating a perfect home for bugs.

4. **Signs of infection**

   The above three strategies will help you prevent an infection. In the unfortunate event you develop a stoma site infection, it's important to treat it quickly before it gets worse and spreads. Look out for the following signs of an infection:

   - Redness
   - Tenderness
   - Thick yellow discharge

- Warmth
- Itching
- Swelling
- Pain on touch.

By preventing stoma site infections or treating them as early as possible, you can significantly contribute to the longevity of your feeding tube.

TUBE HEALTH

Water flushes

Water holds the secret to tube health! It is important to flush your tube with water (room temperature or slightly warmed) before and after each bolus feed or at the start and end of your continuous infusion.

Medication administration

Another secret lies in ensuring the proper administration of medications. Remember to flush with water before and after taking each medication. The common mistake people make is forgetting to flush between each medication. Every single medication should be administered separately, with at least 20ml of water as the ideal practice (Williams 2008). So, for those on multiple medications, the amount of water they consume in a day can add up significantly. It's crucial to discuss the number of medications you take and at what times with your dietitian to find the right balance of water flush frequency and amount for you.

Cap the ports

The third secret is to keep the cap on to close the port when you are not using your tube. This prevents contaminants from entering the tube and helps maintain its integrity and clear colour. Some tubes have one port for everything, while others have two or three ports to separate feeding from medication administration. Ensure that the cap is securely in place to avoid any accidental dislodgement.

Clamp the tube

The fourth secret is to keep your tube clamped when not in use. This prevents unintended liquid backflow from the stomach. If your tube doesn't have a clamp, ask for one.

Regular water flushing, correct medication administration, keeping the cap on and clamping your tube are essential to prevent issues such as tube kinks, cracks, discolouration and sedimentation. You have full control over the health of your tube, and adhering to these guidelines can save you the hassle of an emergency department visit.

DIGESTIVE HEALTH

Digestive health is a key aspect of clinical wellbeing. There isn't one straight definition for a healthy digestive system, but here are some pearls of wisdom around digestive health to get you thinking.

Your mouth matters

Your mouth matters even if you aren't using it for eating. Some key points:

- **Brush:** Brush your teeth twice daily.
- **Dentist:** Visit the dentist regularly to get a general check-up.
- **Moisture:** Keep your mouth moist and fresh with sprays and mouthwashes. Moisture maintains mouth integrity, preventing ulcers and sores from occurring. Our mouth is the gateway to our digestive system. Its health translates to the health of the rest of our digestive tract.
- **Lip balm:** Apply lip balm daily to keep your lips from cracking and potentially getting infected.
- **Saliva:** The normal daily production of saliva varies between 0.5 and 1.5 litres (Iorgulescu 2009). You will likely still produce saliva even if you are tube feeding but how much depends on your hydration

status, what your underlying medical diagnosis is and what medications or treatments you are receiving (Iorgulescu 2009). Make sure you seek support from a speech pathologist on saliva management.

- **Smile:** And, of course, never ever forget that beautiful smile you have. Wear it with tubie pride!

What's your norm?

It's really important to note what is 'normal' for you in terms of bloating and gas build-up. Once you define your baseline norm, be on alert for anything out of the ordinary. For example, some bloating may be normal for you after you have had a tube feed and easily relieved with a bit of movement. But it may not be normal for someone else and can cause them pain, discomfort and sleep deprivation. In such a scenario, introducing some venting (i.e. decompressing air out of the stomach through the feeding tube) 15 minutes before each tube feed may prove successful in proactively controlling gas build-up.

However, this may not be safe to do for everyone, such as those who have had surgery on their digestive system. So, if you think this may be a strategy you'd like to try to help your body expel excess painful gas, it's very important to discuss it with your dietitian and doctor first.

Track the trend

Monitoring trends is crucial. If you experience occasional watery stools once or twice a month without any consistent pattern, it might not be a cause for concern. However, it's essential to remain vigilant for persistent and unusual symptoms that frequently affect your wellbeing, for example, explosive diarrhoea, increased fatigue or changes in your skin hydration or condition.

Should you notice such symptoms, share them with your dietitian. They can work together with you to investigate the underlying causes and explore potential solutions. In some cases, a stool sample analysis might be necessary to identify the root cause. If an infection is detected, a round of antibiotics might be prescribed. Alternatively, if infection is ruled out, medications could be recommended to regulate digestive movement. In cases of malabsorption, where the body struggles to absorb nutrients, enzyme tablets might be suggested to aid digestion.

Early detection and proper management can help address any stool issues and ensure your overall wellbeing.

Look at your poo

In terms of poo, take note of what is normal frequency, consistency and colour for you. Green and yellow watery faeces have different causes and treatment than brown watery faeces. The Bristol Stool Chart is very useful for tracking your stool and communicating any changes to your dietitian (Lewis and Heaton 1997). Google it and use this as your baseline to understand what to look for and report on.

Other symptoms like nausea, hunger pangs and vomiting are all important signs of digestive health. Note how often they are happening and how close they are to your feeding schedule and tell your dietitian.

MEDICATION REVIEW

Unfortunately, many individuals continue taking certain prescription and non-prescription medications for an extended period without undergoing a formal medication review by their doctor or pharmacist. Tube blockages often occur due to incorrect medication administration through a feeding tube or insufficient water flushes (Garrison 2018). To avoid such issues, a helpful guideline is to schedule a medication review every three to six months.

Arrange an appointment with your doctor and ask the following questions:

- "Do I need all these medications I am on?"
- "Am I administering my medications correctly through my feeding tube?"
- "Can I take a liquid form of any of the medications I'm on?"

- "Do any of my medications have the potential to interact with the nutrients in my tube feeding formula?" A good example is insulin which needs to be taken just before nutrition for those who have insulin-dependent diabetes. Your doctor and dietitian will provide guidance on the appropriate medication and nutrition timings.

SKIN, HAIR, NAILS AND EYES

Do not underestimate the impact of nutrition on maintaining the health of your skin, hair, nails and eyes. Although these aspects may not be directly linked to your feeding tube, they can serve as indicators of underlying nutrient deficiencies and other health issues. So, it's essential to remain attentive to any changes that occur in these areas.

Be mindful of new skin irritations, pressure injuries or rashes. Additionally, pay attention to any hair loss, brittle or spoon-shaped nails, or changes in the appearance of your eyes, such as pale colour under your eyelids or difficulty seeing at night. Such signs could potentially signify micronutrient deficiencies or other underlying health concerns that should not be ignored (Reber et al. 2019). Check out Appendix 2 for a pictorial demonstration of what to look out for.

When you notice any of these changes, it's important to discuss them promptly with your doctor and dietitian. By addressing these concerns proactively, you can take necessary steps towards maintaining your overall wellbeing and ensuring that any potential health issues are properly managed. You may need an iron infusion or may be required to take a multivitamin tablet or two.

In summary, clinical signs encompass various aspects of your wellbeing beyond your weight. By monitoring stoma health, tube health, digestive health, stool characteristics and medication considerations, as well as your skin, hair, nails and eyes, you and your dietitian can proactively address any concerns that may arise.

In the next chapter, we will delve into understanding your nutritional needs and what influences them.

Chapter 4

Nourishing your body

BOTH THE AMOUNT AND TYPE of formula you are on are dependent on your nutritional needs. These requirements are based on your underlying medical condition, activity levels, weight goals, organ function and plans for future medical therapy or surgery. Your nutrition needs are continually evolving. Regular review and adjustment of your nutritional intake by a qualified dietitian is necessary.

Let's go through the basic macronutrients and micronutrients you need to be aware of.

FLUID

Adequate hydration is vital for ensuring optimal organ function, promoting healthy digestion and supporting overall health. Generally speaking, 30–35 millilitres per kilogram of body weight per day for an adult is one recommendation for fluid (Institute of Medicine 2005). Other guidelines say 1.6 litres per day for women and 2.0 litres per day for men (Masot et al. 2020). Consult your doctor and dietitian to determine the precise fluid intake that best suits your individual circumstances based on your kidney and heart health as both these organs play pivotal roles in managing fluid build-up and release in the body.

To ensure you are maintaining adequate hydration levels, be aware of the signs of dehydration in the table below.

SIGN	INDICATION OF POTENTIAL DEHYDRATION
Thirst	Feeling thirsty.
Dark urine	Urine is dark yellow or amber.
Less urine output	Urinating less frequently or producing significantly less urine than usual.
Dry mouth and skin	Reduced saliva production, resulting in a dry, sticky feeling in the mouth. Your skin may also feel dry and lack elasticity.

SIGN	INDICATION OF POTENTIAL DEHYDRATION
Fatigue and weakness	A drop in blood volume and blood pressure, leading to feelings of tiredness and weakness.
Dizziness or light-headedness	A drop in blood volume and blood pressure can affect blood flow to the brain.
Rapid heartbeat and breathing	An increase in heart rate and breathing rate.
Sunken eyes	Sunken appearance of the eyes and dark circles around them.
Dry and cool extremities	Hands and feet may feel cooler and appear dry.

While this is not an exhaustive list, it provides a starting point for identifying potential indicators of not having enough fluid. If you notice any of these symptoms or suspect that you may not be consuming enough fluids, discuss this concern with your care team. They can evaluate your situation and make appropriate recommendations to address any hydration issues and optimise your tube feeding regimen.

Fluid intake through your feeding tube encompasses not only the fluid in the formula or homemade blends but also the water flushes around feeds and medication administration. Have a go at calculating how much fluid you are receiving from your feeding regimen – inclusive of water flushes around feeds and medications – and jot it down below, then check it with your dietitian.

I am having _____ ml of fluid in a 24-hour period.

PROTEIN

Protein is a macronutrient that plays a vital role in supporting various bodily functions, including muscle repair and immune system function. The recommended protein intake for adults generally falls within the range of 0.8 to 1.2 grams per kilogram of body weight per day (Paddon-Jones and Rasmussen 2009). However, it's important to note that individual protein requirements can vary based on factors such as your specific medical condition, organ function and nutrition goals. Some medical conditions warrant a protein intake as high as 1.5–2.0 grams per kilogram of body weight per day. To meet someone's protein needs, there are specific high-protein formulas or sometimes protein powders may be added to homemade blends or to water flushes between commercial formula feeds to increase protein intake.

Time your protein

In addition to ensuring you are receiving the total amount of protein per day your body needs, pay attention to how protein is distributed throughout the day. Your body's ability to digest and metabolise nutrition is not only about what you are getting but also when you are receiving it. The science of the impact of meal timing on health is called chrononutrition. Studies suggest that spreading protein intake into regular intervals during the daytime hours can be more effective in supporting the build-up and maintenance of muscle mass (Flanagan et al. 2021).

Whilst these studies have not been performed on people who tube feed, tube-fed adults are definitely not immune to these benefits we are finding in having the 'right' food at the right time. In comparison to a continuous feeding regimen or an overnight feeding regimen, this approach ensures that your body receives protein at the right times during the day – when it is most metabolically active and ready to receive nutrition – therefore promoting optimal utilisation and synthesis of proteins within your muscles.

By addressing your individual protein requirements and ensuring a strategic distribution of protein intake throughout the day, you can optimise muscle maintenance and support overall health while on a feeding tube. Collaborating with your dietitian will help you design a nutrition plan that aligns with your unique circumstances and promotes the best possible outcomes.

CALORIES

When we talk about the number of calories in food, we are referring to the potential energy the food provides to our bodies. When we consume food, our bodies break it down and use its calories to perform various bodily functions, including maintaining body temperature, powering physical activity and supporting essential processes like breathing and organ function. Excess calories that are not used by the body for immediate calorie needs are stored as fat for future use.

Calorie requirements for those who eat through their mouth are not fixed, so nor are they for you as a tube-fed person. Every day differs based on your activity levels, how well you are, your underlying medical diagnosis, how your organs are functioning and more. As such, calories must be adjusted as your circumstances change over time. As you go through different stages of medical treatment, have a new diagnosis or even age, your calorie needs also shift. This is why regular reviews and adjustments of your nutrition plan by a knowledgeable dietitian are important, as they will consider your unique circumstances and tailor your tube feeding plan to meet your specific needs and optimise your overall health.

It's also important to keep your dietitian informed of any changes. If you have recently taken up more hydrotherapy classes or have a new diagnosis from your doctor, let your dietitian know so they can decide whether an adjustment to your calorie intake is necessary.

MICRONUTRIENTS

Checking your micronutrient levels can be a bit tricky because, for various reasons, not all pathology labs offer all the tests. Plus, the levels of these nutrients in your bloodstream don't always give a full picture of what your body actually contains. They can be affected by recent illness or changes in your body fluid status.

The good news is that there are other ways to gauge if you're getting enough micronutrients. Keep an eye out for any signs of deficiency, especially in your skin, hair, nails and eyes, as mentioned in Chapter 3 and Appendix 2. Dietitians often assume that if your weight remains steady and you're meeting your required calories and protein intake, your micronutrient needs are also likely covered. While this might be accurate for the majority of individuals, certain research suggests that this assumption doesn't always apply, particularly in real-life situations where daily formula amounts fluctuate (Breik et al. 2022a; Breik et al. 2022b; McHugh et al. 2023). A study conducted by Tube Dietitian revealed that even when Australian adults relying on tube feeding received their complete prescribed formula, only 75% and 35% of them fulfilled their iron and calcium requirements, respectively (McHugh et al. 2023).

This raises the question: Could micronutrient supplements be necessary regardless of the quantity of formula you're receiving? Our current knowledge about micronutrients isn't comprehensive enough to provide a definitive answer to this question. So, for now, it's wise to consider taking the following actions:

1. Stay watchful and monitor your body for potential signs of deficiency.

2. Get some testing done if you or your dietitian suspect a deficiency or just simply want to check where you are at. There are a few blood tests available in most pathology labs that your doctor can order, like vitamin D, vitamin B12, folate and iron.

3. Chat with your dietitian and doctor. They might recommend a general multivitamin or specific vitamin/mineral supplements to ensure you're getting everything you need, especially if there are any signs of deficiency or if the current formula isn't covering all your needs.

In the next chapter, four common tube feeding challenges will be discussed with some ideas for prevention, as that is always better than cure!

Chapter 5

Rising above challenges

CHALLENGES ARE AN INEVITABLE PART of life, and when it comes to managing a feeding tube, you may encounter various obstacles along the way. However, with proper preparation and knowledge, you can rise above these challenges and ensure a smoother journey. In this chapter, we will explore four tube feeding challenges and provide simple steps to prevent and address them effectively.

CHALLENGE 1: TUBE BLOCKAGE

A blocked feeding tube can be very frustrating. To prevent this issue, it is essential to carry out the following steps:

1. Maintain a regular flushing routine with water.
2. Ensure that medications are administered one

by one through the tube with in-between water flushes.

3. Follow specific instructions provided by your care team regarding tube maintenance. If you don't know what they are, now is the time to ask!

These three prevention steps are relevant to short-term and long-term feeding tubes.

If you encounter a visible blockage, try these tactics at home:

1. Gently massage the area around the blockage by rubbing the tube between two fingers. The warmth from your fingers may move the blockage.

2. Attempt the push-pull technique outlined in Appendix 3. If you haven't been shown how to do this, ask your feeding tube nurse or dietitian to show you.

CHALLENGE 2: TUBE DISLODGEMENT

A tube falling out can be a distressing situation, but it's something you can prepare for. Preventative strategies depend on the type of tube you have. Here are some examples:

1. If you have a nasogastric or nasojejunal tube, make sure it is taped to your cheek with some skin-

friendly medical tape. This will ensure it isn't pulled or tugged at.

2. If you have a gastrostomy or jejunostomy tube, make sure your stoma site stays healthy. If it's a dangler tube, you can wear a belt or lanyard (there are tube feeding specific ones – ask Google!) to avoid it from potentially getting tugged at. If your tube has a balloon as its anchoring device, make sure that its volume is regularly checked by someone in your care team so it doesn't deflate too much and fall out.

If your tube dislodges, immediately cover the stoma site to protect it from any contaminants. Then head to the nearest emergency department with the tube in your hand or bring along a brand-new tube. Keeping a spare tube at home is a wise precaution for such situations. Assume that the hospital closest to your home (or any for that fact!) won't have the exact feeding tube type as your current one. In Chapter 1, you got a glimpse of the various characteristics a tube can have. Carrying a spare can be a smart move given this diversity. Stoma openings can seal up fast, sometimes in less than 24 hours, so it's crucial to get a new tube in quickly to skip the hassle of creating a fresh stoma.

CHALLENGE 3: INTOLERANCE

You can have the perfect formula and perfect regimen and still not be able to stomach it. Tolerance is key for your overall wellbeing. If you notice any new or unusual symptoms after starting a new formula or feeding schedule, it's essential to assess the situation thoughtfully.

Ask yourself the following questions:

- What is my normal state of health and digestion?
- What recent changes have I made to my feeding routine or formula?
- Is this symptom a one-time occurrence or has it been persisting for several days, affecting my quality of life?

Common signs of intolerance may include nausea, vomiting, bloating, diarrhoea or constipation. If you suspect formula intolerance, it's important to consult your dietitian to explore alternative options.

By understanding and being preventative and proactive in managing these common challenges, you can ensure a smoother experience with your feeding tube. If you don't have tangible plans in place now, contact your dietitian and doctor and get them to map some out for you.

CHALLENGE 4: COST

All sections of this book are applicable to anyone with a feeding tube around the globe, except for this section, which is specific to Australia. Regardless, this section might offer valuable insights into potential questions to pose to your dietitian and insurance providers in pursuit of financial assistance even if you live outside Australia.

A recent audit by Tube Dietitian has shown that the average cost of tube feeding for an adult in Australia is $7738 per year (ranging from $1639 to $19,756), with commercial formula making up roughly 72% of the total cost (Young et al. 2023). And the more equipment you use, the more expensive it is. Pump feeding, for example, costs twice as much as syringe bolus feeding (Young et al. 2023). So, home tube feeding is not cheap.

At the time of writing, these are the available financial support options in Australia:

1. State government public health service home tube feeding programs – Depending on the state you live in, the public hospital where you had your tube inserted may cover all the costs associated with formula and equipment with or without a fee. The condition is that ongoing medical and dietetic follow-up must be at that public health service.

2. Australian Government Home Care Packages or Department of Veterans' Affairs support – These programs support older people with more complex needs or those who serve or have served in defence of Australia, respectively, to stay at home. If you meet the eligibility criteria, all costs associated with

tube feeding will be covered. A dietitian can write advocacy letters to ensure you are fully covered for tube feeding costs.

3. The National Disability Insurance Scheme (NDIS) or motor vehicle accident insurance schemes – There are eligibility criteria for both. If you are eligible and approved, all costs will be covered. A dietitian can write advocacy letters to ensure you are fully covered for tube feeding costs.

To date, private health insurance funds haven't exactly stepped up to cover home tube feeding costs. For those who wish to continue with private medical and dietetic follow-ups for their home tube feeding, unfortunately, at this stage you'll be out of pocket. There are ways to reduce your costs such as opting for homemade blended tube feeding rather than commercial formula or transitioning to syringe bolus feeding with minimal equipment needed. Chat with your dietitian, doctor and insurance company. You never know, maybe there is another stream of support that we aren't aware of!

In the next chapter, we will look at the psychological and emotional aspects of the feeding tube experience.

Chapter 6

Supporting the spirit

THE FEEDING TUBE JOURNEY ENCOMPASSES not only the physical aspects but also the psychological and emotional dimensions of your wellbeing. It is essential to acknowledge and address these aspects to ensure a holistic approach to your overall health. In this chapter, we will explore some of the common psychological and emotional experiences that tube-fed adults may encounter during their feeding tube journey and discuss strategies for nurturing your spirit.

LIFE ADJUSTMENT

The transition to using a feeding tube can be a significant adjustment, and it is natural to experience a range of emotions, including fear, hope, frustration, relief and sadness. It is important to give yourself time and space to process these feelings. Understand that it is okay to have mixed emotions and that adjusting to this new aspect of your life takes time. Practise self-compassion and seek support from your care team, loved ones or support groups who can offer empathy and understanding.

Also take comfort from the perspectives of people who are living good and full lives while tube feeding, which you can find online in social media networks (you'll find a few of these listed on the pages to come).

> *"My feeding tube means I'm more likely to focus on my children, I'm more likely to get my PhD, I can go to work and have the mental capacity to analyse important data at work."*
>
> – Tube-fed adult

BODY IMAGE

The presence of a feeding tube may impact your body image and self-esteem. It is normal to have concerns about how others perceive you or how you perceive yourself. Remember that your worth goes beyond your physical appearance. Focus on the strengths and qualities that make you unique. Engage in activities that bring you joy and enhance your self-confidence. Consider speaking with a mental health professional who can provide guidance and support.

*"When I first got my feeding tube, I felt fear,
grief, hope and relief all at the same time."*

– Tube-fed adult

SOCIAL SUPPORTS

Engaging in social interactions and maintaining relationships can sometimes be challenging when you have a feeding tube. Feelings of isolation or worry about how others may react can arise. Open communication is key. Educate your friends, family and close ones about your feeding tube, its purpose and how it positively impacts your life. Most people will respond with understanding and support. Seek out support groups or online communities where you can connect with others who have similar experiences. Sharing your journey with those who can relate can be incredibly empowering and comforting.

*"I've found it far less limiting on what I can do
versus when I'm malnourished and have no
energy. I feel other people around me expect it to
be more complicated or think that it's something
I might be embarrassed to go out with, when I'm
not. It's so much easier to use than they think."*

– Tube-fed adult

COPING MECHANISMS

Building emotional resilience can be beneficial in navigating the ups and downs of the feeding tube experience. Find healthy coping mechanisms that work for you, such as journaling, meditation, engaging in hobbies or seeking therapy. Take time for self-care and prioritise activities that bring you joy and peace. Remember that it is okay to ask for help when needed and to lean on your support network for emotional support.

> *"Having a PEG is not the end of the world. Adapting to it can take time, but eventually it does work. I have travelled to Sydney, Perth and Hobart in the past six months – two trips for work and one for a conference. The flight to Perth was long and I had to eat. I did find something I could manage, and there was ice cream! But I always have a bottle of feed in my bag just in case I don't find a manageable item to eat."*
>
> – Tube-fed adult

CELEBRATE VICTORIES; BE PREPARED FOR SETBACKS

It is important to set realistic expectations for yourself and your feeding tube journey. Recognise that there may be challenges along the way, but also celebrate the small victories and any progress you make. Focus on the improvements in your overall health and wellbeing rather than solely on the presence of the feeding tube. Remind yourself that the feeding tube is a tool that supports your nutrition and health goals.

> *"Now I make the PEG work for me instead of the other way around. I eat lunch (soups etc.) and have started eating breakfast with a modified cereal. I still flush twice a day and have a PEG feed at dinner time. Saves cooking and thinking about what to eat!"*
> – Tube-fed adult

FINDING PURPOSE

Embrace the chance to delve into unexplored aspects of your identity and uncover what truly brings you a sense of purpose and fulfilment. Engage in activities that resonate with your passions and values, allowing them to guide your journey. Through your own experiences, become a source of education and inspiration for others who may be navigating similar paths.

You may find it inspiring to explore the work of Anja Christoffersen, a passionate disability advocate who tube fed for a portion of her life. She founded the Champion Health Agency, a first of its kind 'talent agency' that prioritises lived experience. Its mission is to empower individuals with disabilities and chronic illnesses, and their caregivers, by providing them with meaningful connections and adaptable opportunities to effect transformative change.

Another inspiring story is the work of Yvonne McClaren, founder of the podcast *The No Feeding Tubes Show*. Yvonne was a temporary tube-fed person after a head and neck cancer diagnosis that changed the trajectory of her life. She was determined to get off her PEG tube and used her skills as a qualified chef and writer to document her journey of transitioning off her feeding tube.

Always remember, there is endless value in focusing on your inner wellbeing and cultivating love and connections with those around you.

YOU ARE NOT ALONE

There are several support groups available for individuals with feeding tubes. These support groups provide a space for people to connect, share experiences, exchange information and offer mutual support. At the time of writing, some of the support avenues available for people with feeding tubes include:

1. **ausEE:** This foundation provides resources, support and advocacy for tube-fed people and their families. Founded by a mother of a former tubie, they offer an online community where people can connect, ask questions and share their experiences.

2. **Oley Foundation:** The Oley Foundation is a non-profit organisation that offers support and resources for tube-fed people. They provide a variety of services, including support groups, educational materials and a forum for community interaction.

3. **The Blend magazine:** Melanie Dimmitt, mother of a tubie, is the brilliant editor behind this ingenious online magazine. Be inspired by real-life stories, delicious homemade tube feeding blends and more.

4. **Facebook groups:** There are numerous Facebook groups dedicated to supporting people with feeding tubes. These groups have often been started by tube-fed adults or their carers. They can be specific to certain conditions or open to anyone using a feeding tube. Some examples include 'TubeFed', 'Feeding Tube Australia', 'Real Food 4 Aussie Tubies' and 'Aussie Tubie Mates'.

5. **Pump e-Newsletter:** This is a trusted resource that has successfully connected the tube feeding community for 16 issues and counting since September 2022. All issues can be accessed on the Tube Dietitian webpage in the resources section. The aim of the newsletter is to provide bite-sized home tube feeding information and a sense of community for people and professionals connected to tube feeding.

Joining a support group can be beneficial in providing emotional support, sharing knowledge and finding a sense of belonging within a community of people who understand your experiences with feeding tubes. That said, remember to exercise caution when seeking advice or information from online sources and always consult your dietitian for personalised tube feeding guidance.

> *"Sarah's care family has grown since she went onto tube feeding. As daunting as it was at the start, it has given us great peace of mind knowing that she is well nourished and hydrated. And being able to give her medication when she needs it is now a stress-free procedure."*
>
> – Father of a tube-fed adult

Remember to treat yourself with kindness, reach out for support when necessary and give importance to your emotional and mental wellbeing alongside your physical health.

I trust that this book has been – and will continue to be – a helpful companion on your tube feeding journey, empowering you with the knowledge to take control. For a recap and self-assessment, take a look at Appendix 4, which offers a knowledge check.

Your personal feeding tube journey is yours alone, and by embracing its various aspects, you can nurture a feeling of empowerment and overall wellbeing throughout the entire experience.

References

Bauer J, Biolo G, Cederholm T, Cesari M, Cruz-Jentoft AJ, Morley JE, Phillips S, Sieber C, Stehle P, Teta D, Visvanathan R, Volpi E and Boirie Y (2013) 'Evidence-based recommendations for optimal dietary protein intake in older people: A position paper from the PROT-AGE Study Group', *Journal of the American Medical Directors Association*, 14(8):542–59. doi: 10.1016/j.jamda.2013.05.021

Breik L, Tatucu-Babet OA, Paul E, Duke G, Elliott A and Ridley EJ (2022a) 'Micronutrient intake from enteral nutrition in critically ill adult patients: A retrospective observational study', *Nutrition*, 95:111543. doi: 10.1016/j.nut.2021.111543

Breik L, Tatucu-Babet OA and Ridley EJ (2022b) 'Micronutrient intake from enteral nutrition in critically ill adults: A systematic review of randomised controlled trials', *Australian Critical Care*, 35(5):564–574. doi: 10.1016/j.aucc.2021.09.001

Detsky AS, McLaughlin JR, Baker JP, Johnston N, Whittaker S, Mendelson RA and Jeejeebhoy KN (1987) 'What is subjective global assessment of nutritional status?', *Journal Parenteral and Enteral Nutrition*, 11(1):8–13. doi: 10.1177/014860718701100108

Elia M, Engfer MB, Green CJ and Silk DBA (2008) 'Systematic review and meta-analysis: the clinical and physiological effects of fibre-containing enteral formulae', *Database of Abstracts of Reviews of Effects (DARE): Quality-assessed Reviews* [Internet]. University of York Centre for Reviews and Dissemination (UK). Available from www.ncbi.nlm.nih.gov/books/NBK75630

Flanagan A, Bechtold DA, Pot GK and Johnston JD (2021) 'Chrono-nutrition: From molecular and neuronal mechanisms to human epidemiology and timed feeding patterns', *Journal of Neurochemistry*, 157(1):53–72. doi: 10.1111/jnc.15246

Flood C, Parker EK, Kaul N, Deftereos I, Breik L, Asrani V, Talbot P, Burgell R and Nyulasi I (2021) 'A benchmarking study of home enteral nutrition services', *Clinical Nutrition ESPEN*, 44:387–396. doi: 10.1016/j.clnesp.2021.05.007

Garrison CM (2018) 'Enteral feeding tube clogging: What are the causes and what are the answers? A bench top analysis', *Nutrition in Clinical Practice*, 33(1):147–150. doi: 10.1002/ncp.10009

Griffen C, Hubbard G and Stratton RJ (2023) 'A ready to drink, plant-based oral nutritional supplement is highly complied with, palatable and tolerated in community-based patients at risk of disease-related malnutrition', *Clinical Nutrition ESPEN*, 54:706. doi: 10.1016/j.clnesp.2022.09.722. 'Abstract no. ESPEN22-LB-2147. Presented at ESPEN Congress, Vienna, 3–6 September 2022.

Holdoway A, Page F, Bauer J, Dervan N and Maier AB (2022) 'Individualised nutritional care for disease-related malnutrition: Improving outcomes by focusing on what matters to patients', *Nutrients,* 14(17):3534. doi: 10.3390/nu14173534

Hurt RT, Edakkanambeth Varayil J, Epp LM, Pattinson AK, Lammert LM, Lintz JE and Mundi MS (2015) 'Blenderized tube feeding use in adult home enteral nutrition patients: A cross-sectional study', *Nutrition in Clinical Practice*, 30(6):824–9. doi: 10.1177/0884533615591602

Institute of Medicine (2005). *Dietary Reference Intakes for Water, Potassium, Sodium, Chloride, and Sulfate*. The National Academies Press, Washington. 74–165. doi: 10.17226/10925

Kong F and Singh RP (2008) 'Disintegration of solid foods in human stomach', *Journal of Food Science*, 73(5):R67–80. doi: 10.1111/j.1750-3841.2008.00766.x

Lewis SJ and Heaton KW (1997) 'Stool form scale as a useful guide to intestinal transit time', *Scandinavian Journal of Gastroenterology*, 32(9);920–924. doi: 10.3109/00365529709011203

Iorgulescu G (2009) 'Saliva between normal and pathological. Important factors in determining systemic and oral health', *Journal of Medicine and Life*, 2(3):303–7. PMID: 20112475; PMCID: PMC5052503

Lynch A, Tang CS, Jeganathan LS and Rockey JG (2018) 'A systematic review of the effectiveness and complications of using nasal bridles to secure nasoenteral feeding tubes', *Australian Journal of Otolaryngology*, 1. doi: 10.21037/ajo.2018.01.01

Masot O, Miranda J, Santamaría AL, Paraiso Pueyo E, Pascual A and Botigué T (2020) 'Fluid intake recommendation considering the physiological adaptations of adults over 65 years: A critical review', *Nutrients*, 12(11):3383. doi: 10.3390/nu12113383

McHugh A, Young J and Breik L (11–14 September 2023) 'Iron and calcium requirements for home enteral nutrition patients: An Australian adult' [conference presentation awaiting publication], *ESPEN Congress, Lyon, 2023*. Abstract no. ESPEN23-LB12-T.

Paddon-Jones D and Rasmussen BB (2009) 'Dietary protein recommendations and the prevention of sarcopenia', *Current Opinion in Clinical Nutrition and Metabolic Care*, 12(1): 86–90. doi: 10.1097/MCO.0b013e32831cef8b

Parrish CR and Bridges M (2019) 'Part III Jejunal Enteral Feeding: The Tail is Wagging the Dog(ma). Dispelling Myths with Physiology, Evidence, and Clinical Experience. Nutrition Issues in Gastroenterology', *Practice Gastroenterology*, Series 185. https://med.virginia.edu/ginutrition/wp-content/uploads/sites/199/2019/04/Jejunal-Feeding-Bridges-Parrish-April-2019.pdf

Reber E, Gomes F, Vasiloglou MF, Schuetz P and Stanga Z (2019) 'Nutritional risk screening and assessment', *Journal of Clinical Medicine*, 8(7):1065. doi: 10.3390/jcm8071065

Stajkovic S, Aitken EM and Holroyd-Leduc J (2011) 'Unintentional weight loss in older adults', *Canadian Medical Association Journal*, 183(4):443–449. doi: 10.1503/cmaj.101471

Torquati L, Mielke GI, Brown WJ and Kolbe-Alexander T (2017) 'Shift work and the risk of cardiovascular disease. A systematic review and meta-analysis including dose–response relationship', *Scandinavian Journal of Work, Environment & Health*, 44(3):229–38. doi: 10.5271/sjweh.3700

Walia C, Van Hoorn M, Edlbeck A and Feuling MB (2017) 'The registered dietitian nutritionist's guide to homemade tube feeding', *Journal of the Academy of Nutrition and Dietetics*, 117(1):11-16. doi: 10.1016/j.jand.2016.02.007

Williams NT (2008) 'Medication administration through enteral feeding tubes', *American Journal of Health-System Pharmacy*, 65(24):2347–57. doi: 10.2146/ajhp080155

Young J, McHugh A and Breik L (11–14 September 2023) 'The cost of home enteral nutrition (HEN): an Australian audit' [conference presentation awaiting publication]. *ESPEN Congress, Lyon, 2023*. Abstract no. ESPEN23-LB40-W.

Zheng Y, Manson JE, Yuan C, Liang MH, Grodstein F, Stampfer MJ, Willett WC and Hu FB (2017) 'Associations of weight gain from early to middle adulthood with major health outcomes later in life', *JAMA*, 318:255–69. doi: 10.1001/jama.2017.7092

Appendix 1:
Homemade blended tube feeding

Visit the Tube Dietitian website books page, select the appendix you'd like to download, and enter the code word **TUBE** to access it.

Appendix 2:
Nutrient deficiency signs

Visit the Tube Dietitian website books page, select the appendix you'd like to download, and enter the code word **TUBE** to access it.

Appendix 3:
Home tube feeding

Visit the Tube Dietitian website books page, select the appendix you'd like to download, and enter the code word **TUBE** to access it.

Appendix 4:
Knowledge check

The following 22 questions are derived from this book and can help you assess the state of your tube feeding knowledge and health. Try and answer the questions yourself first. If you come across a question you're uncertain about, consider it a prompt to discuss with your dietitian or doctor.

1. What is the name of the formula you are on and what are its characteristics?

2. What is your feeding regimen mode, method and schedule?

3. What kind of tube do you have?

a. Where does it start?

b. Where does it end?

c. What was the insertion method?

d. Is it a button or dangler?

e. What is the diameter of the tube (French size)?

f. What is holding it in place, the anchoring device?

g. How many ports does it have?

h. Is it ENFit ended?

4. List the tube feeding equipment you use (or need) in a day.

5. Who is in your care team?

6. Have you lost any weight unintentionally?

7. Have you gained any weight unintentionally?

8. When was the last time you had your muscle mass assessed by a health professional?

9. Do you have any water weight on you?

10. What is your stoma's health?

11. What is your tube's health?

12. What is your digestive health?

13. When did you have your last medication review?

14. What is the health of your skin, hair, nails, and eyes?

15. How much fluid are you having in a day?

16. How much protein are you having in a day?

17. How many calories are you having in a day?

18. Are you getting enough micronutrients? Do you need to have a blood test to check?

19. How have you adjusted to life with a feeding tube?

20. How do you feel about your body image?

21. What is your social support network like?

22. What are your coping mechanisms?

Acknowledgements

To my mother and father, your incredible compassion and constant strive for excellence in all aspects of your life have made you the most exceptional parents in the world as well as extraordinary leaders within our society.

To my husband, you are my sanctuary and everlasting spring of encouragement. Your presence in my life is a gift I cherish beyond words.

To Melanie Dimmitt, the word wizard-ess! I will forever be grateful for your kind and thoughtful review of this book.

To Dr Dinesh Palipana, I've been an admirer of your impactful work for a while. Having you write the foreword is an honour beyond measure.

To every person with a feeding tube that I have had the privilege of learning from, you are the inspiration behind this book. Thank you for letting me into your world.

About the author

Lina Breik is an Advanced Accredited Practising Dietitian with over a decade of clinical nutrition experience across various hospitals in Victoria, Australia. She currently serves as the Founding Lead of Tube Dietitian, a business that provides community-based home tube feeding nutrition care and training. Lina's approach to home tube feeding considers the social and emotional aspects of nutrition through a tube. Her aim is to humanise the experience and provide personalised nutrition support that enhances quality of life. Lina's dedication to this cause is exemplified by her current pursuit of a PhD in this specialised area of nutrition.

Connect with Lina!

LinkedIn – www.linkedin.com/in/lina-breik-advapd-4b9a6150/
Twitter – www.twitter.com/TubeDietitian
Website – www.tubedietitian.com
Email – admin@tubedietitian.com

www.ingramcontent.com/pod-product-compliance
Lightning Source LLC
Chambersburg PA
CBHW040758220326
41597CB00029BB/4982